The Ultimate
Eczema Treatment Guide

How to Live Pain Free with Natural
Eczema Treatments and Eczema
Diet Recipes

Mia Soleil

Table Of Contents

Introduction

I want to thank you and congratulate you for purchasing the book, *"Eczema Treatment Guide: How to Live Pain Free with Natural Eczema Treatments and Eczema Diet Recipes."* This book contains natural treatments, strategies and recipes on how to live pain free from eczema and bring healing to your body.

Eczema, or atopic dermatitis, is a medical condition that influences millions of people around the world, predominately experienced by 25% of infants. The constant itchiness and dryness from this skin disease is irritating and painful. The scars it leaves from frequent scratching can scar a person externally as well as internally. People with eczema may feel as though they are on a wild goose chase trying to find the solution to their condition. They are desperate to find relief from the frustration and aggravation of living with eczema.

Eczema may only seem like a minor condition in comparison to the other conditions and diseases that people suffer with. However, people who have experienced eczema know that there is nothing minor about it. The dry, scaly, itchy rash characteristic of eczema wreaks havoc in other areas of life besides the physical. The damage may go deeper than what people can see on the surface. The experiences that come with eczema can also affect the areas of emotional, social, and mental health.

Physically, a simple rash can become inflamed and raw from scratching, developing into an even bigger problem. The larger wound, if in the area of a joint, can make it difficult to move. The constant scratching can cause open wounds which may lead to infections and scarring. In addition, the appearance of eczema is unsightly.

Emotionally, eczema is frustrating, irritating, and exhausting from treatments, appointments, and the lack of results. Embarrassment results when the eczema rash is on areas of the body that the person is not able to cover by clothing. Some people may lose hope of ever finding relief from their condition.

Socially, uneducated people may outcast, bully or isolate a person diagnosed with eczema due to a fear of contamination from an "infectious, contagious disease." These ignorant people are not aware that eczema does not operate in that way. Young children can be especially bad at bullying, teasing and segregating.

Mentally, depression and social withdrawal may occur from an accumulation of all the other areas compounding on top of each other. It's shocking to see a surface rash so deeply affect a person on many levels. Perhaps it will give others compassion for the person with eczema, recognizing that there's a lot more than what meets the eye.

My desire for you is to find encouragement and relief from your eczema through this book. I hope you will find treatments and lifestyle adjustments that you can make in your everyday life to help conquer this beast. Take heart, there is hope. Be strong, persevere, pursue and fight for a life pain free from eczema.

I sincerely thank you again for purchasing this book. I truly hope you enjoy it! Please take some time to stop by and LIKE our Facebook page:

https://www.facebook.com/joypublishing

With gratitude,

Mia Soleil

Mia Soleil

Chapter 1 – What is Eczema?

Eczema is frequently confused with another skin condition known as psoriasis, but the two are simply not the same. To differentiate them, the adult eczema is usually found on the flexor portion of the joints in the body or those parts on the inner side of a joint that can reduce in size or area due to flexing. Alternatively, psoriasis is not commonly found in those parts.

Eczema is a kind of dermatitis which refers to the inflammation of the outermost layer of the skin or the epidermis. It is a condition in which certain portions of the skin become irritated and scabrous. The skin can break out in blisters that cause itchiness and bleeding. This may be due to the skin's reaction to an irritant medically referred to as eczematous dermatitis. However, more commonly the condition may emerge without evident environmental or external cause.

This skin problem usually begins during the early years but it can also start later in life. Eczema is typically identified with dry, severely itchy, red-colored patches on the skin. Because some people, especially the young kids, cannot avoid scratching when the patches of skin become itchy, they tend to have rashes.

Chapter 2 - Causes of Eczema

There must be some sort of trigger that brings about the eruption of the irritating red-colored lesions commonly observed among people who are suffering from eczema. For instance, a break out of contact dermatitis may have been caused by something as outwardly safe as being dressed in garments made of coarse fabric. These rough clothing may be made of wool or other materials like it. Moreover, cigarettes or tobacco, soaps with strong chemicals, bleach, smoke, animal fur or hair, and other chemical substances can trigger the break out of eczema. This can particularly occur among little children who are vulnerable to this type of skin condition.

The major causes of majority of the usual types of eczema are hereditary in nature. One parent or both of them may have experienced this skin problem due to allergic reactions like runny nose and asthmatic attacks. This kind of susceptibility can be passed on from one generation to the next.

Even if eczema is usually a hereditary condition, a flare-up is also contingent to the type of condition a patient has.

Atopic eczema or infantile eczema – This is the most prevalent form that is known to be hereditary. It is usually seen among kids whose immune system may be severely reacting to certain triggers like flakes of the skin, animal hair or fur, dust mites, pollen, among others. Exposure can result to inflamed, chafed, and itchy skin.

Contact dermatitis – This is brought about by contact with any irritant which can set off skin eruptions.

Xerotic eczema – This is not a common type and affects the elderly. It is caused by skin dryness that usually occurs at a certain season of the year. The skin becomes dry and ultimately breaks out.

Other types

Neurodermatitis – This type manifests with inflamed red-colored lichen eczema typically caused by continuous scratch and rub actions.

Dyhidrosis - This type of eczema is concentrated on the palms, the sides of the fingers, and the soles of the feet. It feels itchier during the night.

Venous eczema – This commonly occurs among individuals aged above fifty years old whose circulation is impeded.

Discoid eczema – This condition aggravates during extreme cold weather and is characterized by lesions on the lower portion of the leg.

Determining the Cause

Allergy testing under medical supervision is a wide-ranging method that can precisely isolate the cause of an eczema problem. Aside from determining one's allergies, this kind of test will also determine the personal reactions of a particular individual to certain allergens like molds, pollens, or drugs. This test will be able to indicate what it is you are exactly allergic to. This might take some time before results are obtained. The medical practitioner working on you might have found numerous allergens which you might be reacting to; hence, the process may not be completed as fast as you want it to.

Taking this test is not only beneficial for exactly determining the kinds of food products or substance in them that you are reacting against. This will also determine any factor in the environment that may also be triggering your eczema. Among these environmental factors are smoke, dust mites, pollen, and some chemicals found in hygiene and cleaning products.

Naturopaths have been known to request blood work for their patients in order to determine whether there are specific foods that are triggering the eczema. It is believed by doctors that the health of the digestive system indicates the health of the entire body. Eczema can simply be the symptom of a greater cause that is occurring in the digestional tract. Once a patient brings healing to their digestive system through treatments and diet, the eczema takes care of itself.

Chapter 3 – Symptoms of Eczema

Among young children including babies, eczema manifests as dry pigmented patches on the forehead, the cheeks, neck, head, upper arms, and legs. For these kids, their condition will progressively be relieved while they are growing up. Hence, kids who had eczema while they were infants and toddlers will no longer suffer from it as they grow into adulthood. There are more than a few factors which can bring about this skin problem even among adults who have not had eczema for a number of years. As this occurs among adults, the dry pigmented skin will usually be found on the inner part of the elbows and knees, and less common on the ankles.

However, the problem can also break out to present numerous of characteristics that are typically observed in eczema that affects children. People should not worry even if this is a chronic problem and there has been no known absolute cure for it because it is not life threatening. Moreover, there are numerous methods to prevent and manage a break out. However, since the major cluster among those that are affected is comprised of young kids who have difficulty with avoiding scratching, it is typical for them to break the skin which results to vulnerability to infection and development of other skin problems.

Suggestions

> ➤ Getting an allergy test must be taken into account. This kind of test may sometimes be time-consuming and also painful. However, it is important to determine what has

caused the eczema symptoms to come out. Possible causes include carpets, animals, food, and foliage.

➢ When your hands are affected and it is difficult to do regular household tasks like washing, you can use hand gloves. Smear your hands with moisturizer and some coconut oil. Don the gloves and leave them on for an hour and take them off for an hour also. Apply the lotion and coconut mixture on the hands every time you will wear and take off the gloves.

➢ For some people, an allergy test can be cumbersome and sometimes costly. If this is the case, you can jot down all the things you have eaten, worn, and done on a certain day. For instance, you can write in your journal that you ate fruits, wore a knitted blouse, and visited a nursery in your local plant store or used a certain product that might have triggered your eczema. Make a note of the way you felt during this day and also note how many times you felt itchy during the day and for how many days this itchiness continued. In the long run, you will be able to point out certain patterns related to your condition.

Chapter 4 – Natural Treatments

Lifestyle modification

- *Healthier diet*

It is imperative to bear in mind that whenever there is a health issue like eczema, the skin remains as the biggest organ functioning to eliminate waste products from the body. This indicates that anything introduced inside the body may also manifest externally when the skin expels waste. It is a fact that a person's diet has a lot to do with the skin's wellbeing. Hence, certain minor modifications can result to major improvements to a case of eczema. Concentrate on ingesting food products that are good for the stomach and the liver, and eradicate processed foods and those high in gluten from the diet.

Replace a typical diet with a more nutritious one comprised of raw vegetables, fruits, seeds, and nuts. Use grass-fed beef, pork, and chicken instead of the usual meat products in the market. Eat lots of omega-3 fatty acid-rich foods like chia, salmon, hemp seed, and walnuts. As much as possible, remove gluten from your choices of food since it can bring about eczema. Steer clear of cereals, bread, pasta, and other processed foods with high carbohydrate content.

- *Wheat based food products need to be avoided.*

Food items such as biscuits, breads, and other baked products have wheat flour that is typically loaded with gluten. Like other wheat based and commonly baked products, gluten is known to trigger eczema break outs. People need to try out certain changes in their diet like steering clear of gluten-based foods for some time. Drinks like caffeinated substitutes, root beer, and the common beer may have grain and yeast. The latter ingredient is another substance found in majority of bread products. Yeast is a type of fungus that is believed to cause eczema. You can experiment by avoiding foods that contain this ingredient just to see if it is one of the triggering factors of your eczema flare-up.

- *Acidic fruits are not recommended for individuals who are suffering from eczema.*

According to research studies, eating acidic fruits like currants, cranberries, and blueberries can heighten the level of skin generation affected by eczema. Glazed fruits and canned fruit products may also cause a flare-up. Mainly due to the preservatives used and the glazing or canning procedures that are most typically used.

- *Dairy products including soy have to be removed from the diet.*

Milk from cows is probably a major food product that causes eczema. This is the reason it needs to be eradicated from the diet for at least two weeks to observe if there will be any changes. Milk from cows has acid and usually contains chemicals and hormones which adversely affect the immune system and worsen the skin condition.

Unfermented soy products contain enzyme inhibitors that can interfere with healthy digestion. If you chose to use soy products, choose fermented products such as tempeh, miso and tamari sauce.

Lots of products can be used to replace milk that comes from cow. There are milk products with the same creaminess that are sourced from goat, sheep, and buffalo. If you prefer milk that does not come from any animal, almond, coconut, hemp, rice and oat milk are great substitutes. It must be noted that even if removing dairy products and milk can help ease symptoms, it is imperative to obtain calcium and nutrients from other sources like dark green leafy vegetables. Another good alternative is to take supplements.

Take supplements with natural components. If at all possible, people would obtain all their required nutrients and vitamins from their daily diet. However, this seldom happens in real life. Fortunately, there are ample nutritional supplements in the market that can fight against eczema. These include:

> Fatty acids. They relieve skin dryness and diminish inflammation, which makes them effective in managing eczema. A supplement that has Omega 3, 6, and 9 is the best option. Choose a good quality fish oil since many companies do not properly remove the alcohol that is used in the production process. Make sure that there is no wheat, dairy or yeast in the oil. The best products are usually found in a specialty health foods store or through a naturopath.

> Vitamins A, D, and E. These fat soluble vitamins have amalgamated benefits for the skin that are remarkable. They help in keeping the skin hydrated, enhance its

texture, increase production of collagen, and shield it from harmful free radicals.

➢ Supplements with gamma-linolenic acid (GLA). GLA is a fatty acid that is included in borage oil, black currant oil, and evening primrose oil. GLA relieves inflamed skin and has the capacity to adjust the skin's lipid balance.

- *A diet rich in alkaline foods*

On a pH scale, the body is healthiest at 7.36. This means that the body functions best when it is slightly alkaline. Therefore, a diet predominantly rich in alkaline foods is very important. When the body is acidic, the body works hard to restore its alkaline state. The body will do whatever it takes to bring this balance, even if it means taking nutrients from other areas of the body. When our body is in an acidic state, which the mass population will often find itself, diseases and sicknesses are invited into the body. When there is garbage, rats come. The body is capable of healing itself when it is naturally alkaline. Unwanted weight starts to shed itself, skin starts to clear up, fatigue disappears and many other positive changes occur when we focus on eating more alkaline than acidic. The alkalinity and acidity of food are referring to the residual ash that occurs when the food is broken down in the body. Just because a lemon is acidic does not mean it is acidic on the pH scale. The alkaline list consists of primarily fruits and vegetables with protein products including eggs, almonds, and chicken. Commonly enjoyed foods like grain, dairy, and beef, pork, and lamb are found on the acidic list.

- *Wear clothing that do not irritate the skin.*

Clothing is worn to cover and protect the skin. But it brushes and rubs on the skin, which for some people can cause chafing. Others observe their eczema worsening during winter when they use more layers of clothes. For some affected individuals, the worse the eczema becomes, the more they want to be covered. The more it is covered, the more the irritation gets worse. As a result, a vicious cycle occurs. This may be addressed by choosing the appropriate clothes.

Choose loose-fitting or unrestricting clothing and keep away from prickly and irritating cloth material. Smooth fabrics are made from cotton, bamboos, and silk. During exercise use appropriate sportswear designed for comfort and to keep cool in hot weather. This will keep you from perspiring too much which can make eczema worse. In addition, check your detergent for washing clothes. It should not leave even a tiny bit of residue on the clothes that are known to cause break outs in eczema. Natural powder or a biological brand is a better option.

- *Diminish stress*

Eczema and other problems of the skin have been firmly associated with physical and psychological stress. Hence, working on diminishing stress can be really helpful. It isn't realistic to eliminate all stress from our life. However, learning healthy coping mechanisms will benefit your skin and other areas of your life greatly. Alternative methods like the use of visualization and hypnosis as therapeutic technique have been recommended to reduce stress; however, less difficult stress relieving techniques can be integrated into one's activities of daily living.

17

➢ Simple meditation. A few minutes daily to remain at a serene location within the house or outside with eyes closed, and concentrated on one's breaths can be immensely beneficial for physical and mental wellbeing. Some people murmur a calming mantra while meditating. Other physical activities like yoga can provide similar healthy outcomes.

➢ Playing and listening to music. This activity has been shown to lower blood pressure and lessen anxiousness which makes it an excellent solution to manage stress. Relaxing music like the classical type or nature sounds can be very soothing. Other people prefer singing along with the type of songs they like to help them relax and feel good.

➢ Adequate sleep. Not getting enough sleep can cause severe stress. Hence, you need to have seven up to eight hours of sleep on a nightly basis to diminish stress. If you are a light sleeper, have a soothing bath prior to going to bed. The room where you sleep must be cool and all light sources switched off. Discontinue watching a television or any form of computer screen at least an hour, ideally two, before going to sleep.

- *Use non-irritating hygiene products*

The shampoos and soaps you use can have immense effect on your skin's condition, so it is vital to recognize the components of the products you use. Bear in mind that the more a product is made of natural components, the less harsh it will be on a skin vulnerable to eczema. It is imperative to steer clear of deodorizing and antibacterial items since they can cause dryness of the skin.

- ➢ Do not use soaps and shower products with scents and dyes. They may appear attractive and fragrant but they are definitely filled with irritating compounds that can cause dryness to the skin.

- ➢ Do not choose items with sodium lauryl sulfate. Certain soaps and shampoos use this chemical as foaming substance. This chemical is also an ingredient in cleaning products for floors and vehicles. Therefore, it can be extremely harsh on human skin because it destroys the natural proteins in the skin. When this happens, the skin becomes more susceptible to toxic substances.

- ➢ Parabens is also a group of chemicals that need to be avoided. This is typically found in hygiene products like body scrubs, lotions, shampoos, and hair conditioners. They have been found to cause unfavorable effects on the skin and other issues affecting health.

- • *Use a device to increase humidity in the room.*

When you have dry air, this can worsen eczema. It causes the skin to peel or become flaky due to dryness. This can be managed by using an air humidifier that functions to increase humidity in the air and moisture to the skin. Devices like this for home use can be connected to a heating system.

However, there are also ways to increase humidity without having to purchase this appliance. You can place indoor plants like ferns to serve as natural humidifiers in the house or in your room. Another way is to fill a container with water under a source of heat. Evaporation of this liquid can increase air humidity in the room.

- *Use warm water less often when taking a bath.*

When you take a shower, it can feel relaxing particularly to dry skin. But it must be noted that frequent bathing can take away the skin's natural moisture which can result to worsening an eczema condition. Therefore, if you have this skin problem, you can lower the water temperature when taking a shower. Do not stay in the bath too long. A fifteen to twenty minutes bath is fine.

➢ Remember to apply an ample amount of lotion, cream, oil-based product following your bath before drying off in order to more effectively lock in moisture. Use your hands to remove excess moisture applied on the skin.

➢ In addition, make certain that you have dried yourself completely. Also make sure you do not rub the towel too harshly on the skin so as not to aggravate its condition.

Natural Remedies

- *Aloe Vera*

The thick liquid substance from this plant has always been known to manage skin conditions such as burns or wounds. It has relieving qualities that is great for eczema. It can moisturize the skin at the same time relieves itching.

> ➢ When taking the sap from an aloe vera plant, break off a leaf and force out the thin liquid substance inside. Apply this on the skin and leave it on to be absorbed. The rest of the leaf may be refrigerated for other purposes.

> ➢ It is recommended to use an aloe vera plant instead of getting gel products and lotions with aloe vera as an ingredient. These skin moisturizing products in the market use other components aside from aloe vera that may aggravate eczema.

> ➢ There has been no reported side effect in using aloe vera straight from the plant. It can be used regularly.

- *Chamomile*

Since chamomile acts to relieve inflammation and itchiness, it has been an accepted natural treatment for eczema.

> ➢ With chamomile, you can make tea by adding its flowers to boiling water for fifteen minutes. Drain and remove the flowers from the liquid. Using a clean piece of cloth,

immerse this in the liquid and use it on the skin to relieve itchiness and inflammation. Apply the warm cloth ten to fifteen minutes.

➢ Essential oils with chamomile can also be used to relieve eczema. The oil can be applied on the skin or add it to a tub filled with warm water for bathing. Chamomile is effective; however, some individuals have hypersensitivity. Apply a little on a small part of your skin to test for any reaction.

- *Calendula lotion*

Extract from the calendula flower is used as an active ingredient when making ointments, creams, soaps, oils, and lotions for the skin. It can relieve inflammation and pain. Products in health food outlets are known to have higher amounts of pure calendula and other components that are good for the skin. There have been no reported ill effects in using these products.

- *Coconut oil*

The virgin coconut oil variety is very effective as a moisturizing agent for the skin. When it is cold pressed, it looks solid but will immediately liquefy and applied on the affected portions of the body. When you say cold pressed, it means that it had gone through process at temperatures less than 116°. In this temperature, the mineral, enzymes, and nutrients of the oil can be preserved or maintained. .

- *Warm bath*

A warm bath with additional ingredients to help manage eczema can be extremely effective in relieving pain and itching. Bear in mind that when hot water is used, this can worsen the skin problem. Just maintain a tepid or warm temperature.

Additions to the bath may include:

➢ One tablespoon of baking soda is a great addition to the water to relive itchiness of the skin.

➢ Raw oatmeal or fine oatmeal may be drizzled into the water to relax the skin. The finely ground variety is really used for bathing in.

➢ A half cup of bleach may be mixed into the water. This is to eradicate the bacteria that remain on the skin's epidermis and in turn prevent the spread of eczema. This solution has been standardized according to bath tub size used in the United States. Water is filled up to the level of the drainage openings. If it is your first time to use this dilution, you may begin with ¼ cup. It is recommended to begin with ¼ cup of regular 6% bleach and never use more than ½ cup of it. Be aware that there are certain concentrated types in the market. If this is your bleach, the ratio and proportion to be used is different.

➢ *Evening primrose oil*

This has been used as a natural alternative to manage eczema because it is known to contain an uncommon fatty acid called gamma-linolenic acid. It helps to nurture the skin by lessening inflammation. It is typically taken by mouth as a supplement.

- *Sweet almond oil*

This is also used to manage eczema because it has oleic acids and ursolic acids. These components help in repairing damaged skin and reducing inflammation. It is used to moisturize the entire body. Some people apply it all over the skin before they shower or immerse in a bath. It helps to produce a kind of protection that prevents dryness caused by using hot water for bathing.

- *Olive oil*

Olive oil has a great moisturizing effect. Place a mixture of sugar and olive oil combined in equal amounts on the skin's affected parts. Carefully remove the sugar on the skin using a clean moist cloth.

- *Apple cider vinegar*

Combine apple cider vinegar 50% that is not filtered with 50% water. Apply on areas with eczema two times daily until it turns dry. Coconut oil may be used for moisturizing dry skin.

Alternative treatments

Among alternative treatments include acupuncture, homeopathy, and hypnosis along with others. Some people have reported these methods helped them manage their skin problem since stress is alleviated during sessions. For people who have tried everything, these may be good alternatives for treating eczema.

Chapter 5 – The Power of Hydration

You may not be familiar with this natural treatment for eczema but it is far more essential than any other treatment presented in this book. This topic is so foundational, so crucial, so revolutionary, that it deserves to have a chapter of its own. It is of utmost importance for people to understand the water they are consuming on a daily basis in order to nourish their bodies.

Since our body is composed of 75% water, it is imperative to keep your body hydrated. However, not all water is created the same. While water, regardless where you find it, has the basic chemical compounds of H_2O, the structure of water is not created equal. Depending where you live, your tap water may actually not be the best source water. World wide, bottled watered is generally a popular alternative. However, people aren't aware of the damage that is being done to not only the environment but the human body. When considering our water source, there are some factors to consider such as its oxidation rating and its pH level.

First of all, it's important to note that plastic water bottles are one of the world's top pollutants. 1 out of 6 plastic bottles are actually recycled. This poses huge implications on the environment on many different levels. While this does not directly impact eczema, the long term repercussions can pose a lot of damage to our health and environment.

That being said, the plastic bottles that bottled water come in leech harmful chemicals into the contained water that contribute to raising estrogen levels in the human body. Due to the process of time that spans production, packaging and transportation, the bottled water resides in its plastic bottle for lengthy periods of time. Therefore, the plastic chemicals have a longer window of time to leak into our water source. These are chemicals that should not be introduced into our body since they wreak havoc and create long term health implications.

Furthermore, bottled water and tap water have a higher positive oxidation rating which is correlated to free radicals in the body. These water sources are contributing to the problem of diseases and cancers rather than helping prevent them. It's horrifying to discover that the tap water in my city, which is considered top quality, is actually worse than the 7-Up soda in relation to its oxidation rating. 7-Up was at least +400 while the tap water was over +600! Bottled water was near equivalent to 7-Up and power drinks in terms of its oxidation rating.

Besides the oxidation rating factor, it is essential to take into account the pH level of water. The pH level in our water source is incredibly important, especially when we are looking at ways to heal eczema. Bottled water falls below neutral with 5/6 acidity. An acidic pH level is not good considering our body is 7.365 alkaline. Tap water's ph level will depend on where you live. In my area, where water is top quality, tap water is neutral at 7 on the pH scale. In some areas, the water is neutralized to reduce rusting of the water pipes (isn't that nice?).

In addition, chlorine is added to remove bacteria from the water since water poisoning is one of the top causes of death in the world. In the summer, the city increases the chlorine level to accommodate for the hotter climate. I don't recall getting any notification about this from my city to warn me. Consequently, the chlorine in the water is instantly absorbed into the body which poses problems with our liver. If we shower in this water, the chlorine dries out the skin, which further exasperates the problem of eczema.

The beauty of alkaline water is that is supports the alkaline balance in our body. When our body is in an alkaline state, it functions the way it was intended to. Eczema naturally disappears because the body is in harmony. Remember that skin is an indicator of internal health. When our body is in an acid state, it shows itself in our skin. The body is smart. It will take nutrients from other areas of the body and do whatever it needs to do to maintain its alkaline state. Taking this information into consideration, the fastest way to heal eczema is to bring the body into an alkaline state. This can quickly be achieved by drinking alkaline water. The next best thing is consuming a diet rich in alkaline foods – predominately plant based foods.

Alkaline water is 8.5-9.5 alkaline and hydrates the body more efficiently than bottled or tap water. In addition, it detoxifies the body by neutralizing the acids and removing the toxic waste. One of the best sources of alkaline water on the market is Kangen water.

Kangen water uses a filter system that is attached to your sink in order to filter the water and create an alkaline pH level. In addition, the system ionizes the tap water through electrolysis which produces a negative oxidation rating. That means it's an antioxidant and takes away the free radicals from the body. Furthermore, Kangen water can be used for cooking, beauty and cleaning. It's shocking to see all the pesticides and chemicals that wash off your vegetables after you use Kangen water to clean them.

When you get your hands on Kangen water, try a full body water transfusion. Drink 1 ounce for every pound of body weight a day. For an average 140 lb woman, that's about a gallon a day! Drink the same amount for 21 days and watch your body heal itself from the inside out. It's incredible! This may be the single most difference maker for you in the healing of your eczema.

Chapter 6

Anti-Eczema Recipes

- *Salmon and Garden Salad*

Some people who have eczema may be hypersensitive to sea foods like fish. If you do not have any allergy, omega-3 fatty acids rich salmon is very effective in controlling eczema symptoms. Aside from fatty acids, salmon has a type of carotenoid that gives its pinkish color and is a strong antioxidant. Carrots, radishes, and lettuce with long crisp leaves used in this salad provide ample vitamin C and are very effective in managing the skin condition. This salad recipe serves 2.

Ingredients:

1 head lettuce with long crisp leaves

5 ounces thinly cut smoked salmon

2 pieces diced tomatoes

4 thinly cut radishes

1 sliced carrot

½ peeled and sliced cucumber

Extracted juice of half lemon

1 teaspoon peeled and minced ginger

1 teaspoon olive oil

Procedure:

1. Place the washed lettuce leaves on a large plate.

2. Arrange the salmon, radishes, tomatoes, cucumber, and carrots on top of the lettuce.

3. Combine olive oil, ginger, and extracted juice.

- Drizzle dressing over the salad.

- *Carrot Muffins*

The main ingredients for these muffins are carrots. They are free of gluten and so are best for individuals who are sensitive to gluten. Aside from carrots, the recipe also includes flaxseeds. This combination is effective in preventing inflammation of the skin. This recipe makes 12 muffins.

Ingredients:

1 cup of rice milk

1 raw egg

1 tablespoon grounded flaxseeds

1 teaspoon Xanthan gum

1 teaspoon cinnamon

1 cup grated carrots

¼ cup raisins

¼ cup brown sugar

½ teaspoon salt

2 cups flour (gluten-free)

3 ½ teaspoons baking powder (gluten-free

4 tablespoons coconut oil

Procedure:

1. Preheat oven to 400°F or 200°C.
2. Line a muffin tin with 12 paper liners or lightly grease with shortening or cooking spray.
3. Beat the egg in a small bowl. Add the milk and coconut oil. Stir until wet ingredients are combined.
4. Sift dry ingredients together in a large bowl. Make a "well" or crater in the center of the dry ingredients.
5. Pour the wet ingredients all at once into the center of the well in the dry ingredients. Using a rubber spatula or wooden spoon, gently stir together and mix just until dry ingredients are moistened. Make sure not to mix too much or your muffins will have peaks and tunnels.
6. Add in the raisins and grated carrots. Stir gently to evenly distribute.
7. Fill muffin cups with the batter 1/3 full. Make sure to wipe away any spilled batter.
8. Bake for twenty minutes. A toothpick inserted into the center of the muffin should come out clean and dry.
9. Remove muffins from muffin tin and cool on cooling rack.

- *Carrot and Beet Salad*

Combined carrots and beets provide an excellent natural remedy for eczema. These vegetables are filled with nutrients that are good for the skin. The recipe also features ginger root which is a good anti-inflammatory.

Ingredients:

½ cup of grated carrots

½ cup of peeled and grated beets

½ teaspoon of minced ginger

1/8 teaspoon sea salt

1 tablespoon extra virgin olive oil

2 tablespoons of apple juice

Procedure:

1. Mix the carrots and beets in a bowl.
2. Combine the olive oil, apple juice, ginger, and salt.
3. Sprinkle olive oil mixture on the salad mix and carefully toss.

- *Healthy Omelet*

If a person with eczema does not have an allergy to eggs, an omelet with red onions and capers can be great for inflamed skin. These two ingredients contain bioflavonoid with anti-inflammatory, antihistamine, and antioxidant properties.

Ingredients:

1 chopped red onion

¼ teaspoon salt

1 ½ tablespoon of water

2 tablespoons extra virgin olive oil

3 teaspoon capers

4 eggs

Procedure:

1. Fry onion in a pan with olive oil until it turns golden brown.
2. Combine beaten egg, salt, and water in a bowl.
3. Add in the capers and pour the mixture in the pan with cooked onions.
4. Turn the omelet when done and then place on a serving plate.

- *Carrot and Beet Soup*

This soup makes use of vegetables with nutrients that help protect the skin. Similar to the salad recipe, this also includes fresh ginger root with potent anti-inflammatory action.

Ingredients:

1 cup chopped onion

1 tablespoon oil

1 pound diced carrots

1 clove minced garlic

1 minced ginger

3 peeled and diced beets

6 cups vegetable stock

Procedure:

1. Sauté the onion in a pan until golden brown.
2. Add in ginger and garlic.
3. In two minutes, toss in the carrots and beets.
4. Pour the vegetable stock.
5. Lower the heat and allow to it simmer.
6. Cover the pan until the vegetables are done within 25 minutes.
7. Puree the soup one batch at a time. Season to taste and garnish with cilantro.

- *Pudding with Chocolate Flavoring*

Some people who suffer with eczema cannot tolerate chocolate. However, it is still possible to enjoy its rich sweetness and texture through this pudding recipe. It is made with carob flour that has a flavor similar to cocoa. Aside from the carob flour, this recipe includes dates and millet grain which are also ideal for people with hypersensitivity.

Ingredients:

1/3 cup chopped dates

½ teaspoon vanilla

1/8 teaspoon salt

¾ cup of water

1 1/3 cups of freshly cooked millet

2 tablespoons of carob flour

Procedure:

1. Combine the dates and water and blend until it reaches a smooth consistency.
2. Place this mixture in a saucepan and boil.
3. Turn off the heat and put all the ingredients in the pan.
4. Mix until smooth.
5. Refrigerate the pudding and serve.
   Oatmeal Muesli

This is a popular breakfast food made with uncooked oats. This recipe includes red grapes with antioxidants that work to start of synthesis of collagen and in turn enhances skin. This recipe is beneficial for people with eczema.

Ingredients:

½ cup of puffed buckwheat from a local food store

½ cup chopped dried apples

1 cup diced pears

1 cup sliced red grapes

1 ½ cups of rolled oats

2 teaspoons ground cinnamon

3 tablespoons brown sugar

Rice milk

Procedure:

6. Preheat oven to 32°F.
7. Place the oats on a baking tray.
8. Toast this in the preheated oven for ten minutes. Stir the oats from time to time. Make sure not to burn the toasted oats.
9. Take this out from the oven allow to cool.
10. Place the oats in a bowl and pour water to be soaked until the following day.
11. Add in the buckwheat, apples, cinnamon, and sweetener to the oats. Mix well.
12. Serve with grapes and pears on top, and rice milk.

- *Fruits Smoothie*

This smoothie recipe is filled with anti-inflammatory phytonutrients and antioxidants. It has quercetin, a flavonoid that is effective for eczema because of its anti-inflammatory effects. This smoothie also includes flaxseeds and raspberries which contain omega-3 fatty acids.

Ingredients:

1 sliced ripe and frozen banana

1 cup raspberries

1 tablespoon ground flaxseeds

1 cup of grain milk from rice

Procedure:

1. Mix the banana, raspberries, flaxseeds, and rice milk together in a blender until consistency is smooth.
2. Add more fruits or other garnishing on top and serve.

- *Asparagus with Quinoa Noodles*

This is a tasty noodle recipe at the same time it has loads of antioxidants that is beneficial in combating eczema.

Ingredients:

½ tablespoon of sugar

1 tablespoon olive oil

1 tablespoon soy sauce

2 bundles of washed and cut asparagus

3 teaspoons minced ginger

3 ½ tablespoons vegetable stock

12 ounces quinoa noodles (dried)

Procedure:

1. Cook the noodles in a large pot of boiling water. Check package for cooking time. Drain and set aside.
2. Over medium heat, stir-fry the ginger and garlic.
3. After two minutes, add the bite sized asparagus.
4. When asparagus is tender, add the remaining ingredients. Cook sauce for 2-3 more minutes or until sauce is heated through.
5. Pour asparagus and sauce over top the bed of noodles.
   - *Vegetable Soup*

The main ingredients in this vegetable soup are the watercress and winter pea. Since centuries ago, households have used watercress as treatment for certain complaints in terms of health. It has anti-inflammatory and cleansing properties that help to relieve eczema.

Ingredients:

1 large sized potato

1 clove of garlic

1 chopped onion

6 cups of chicken stock

3 ounces water cress

30 ounces water peas

Salt and pepper

Procedure:

1. Pound the garlic and set aside. Leave the pounded garlic for about five to ten minutes for it to maximize its beneficial effects.
2. Peel and cut the potato and onion.
3. In a saucepan, add in two to three tablespoons of chicken stock and then add the onion and garlic.
4. Add the potato pieces and pour the remaining chicken stock into the saucepan.
5. As soon as it boils, allow to simmer until potato chunks are tender.

6. Put the winter peas in the soup and simmer for a few minutes.

7. Add the watercress.

8. When finished, turn off the heat, leave the soup, and let it cool down.

9. Place the soup in batches in a blender until smooth. Season it with salt and pepper according to your taste.

Conclusion

Thank you again for purchasing this book.

I hope this book was able to help you find treatments and strategies on how to live pain free from eczema.

The next step is to apply these strategies and make changes to your diet. It's shocking how the food we eat has such profound affects on the body...especially sugar. I'm amazed by how much better my body feels after cutting sugar out of my diet for even 2 weeks. It has been incredibly difficult for me to do, but I've come to a point of desperation which propels me to make the changes necessary.

Finally, please remember to check out our Facebook page in order to find other resources and upcoming promotions:

https://www.facebook.com/joypublishing

Sincerely,

Mia Soleil

Preview Of "Guide to Pain Management: How to Achieve Pain Relief and Live Pain Free for Life"

Pain and the Body

When you cut yourself, blood oozes out and there's a sharp pain that follows. If you have a migraine, you feel a chronic throbbing pain in your head. If you are burnt, pain is intensely unbearable. These are different scenarios where a person undergoes a painful experience. Pain in varying degrees of intensity and frequency is identified. The definition of pain, however, is out of the question.

What is pain?

Pain is a complex stimulus. There is no exact definition because it is an entirely subjective sensation. It is the foremost reason why people seek medical attention. Pain tells you that something is wrong or damaged. The International Association for the Study of Pain defines it as "an unpleasant sensory and emotional experience associated with actual or potential tissue damage or described in terms of such damage".

In actual context, pain is not always associated with physiological processes. Medical attention can identify and treat physical pain, but there's also another kind of pain which is really hard if not impossible to treat through medical means...emotional pain. So what is pain? Pain, to put it simply, is far more than neural transmission and sensory transduction. It is a complex mixture of emotion, sensation, culture, experience and spirit.

How does the body react to pain?

Pain perception or nociception is the process where a painful stimulus is signaled and relayed to the central nervous system from the point of origin. It is entirely different when compared to normal stimuli like touch, ordinary pressure and temperature. When the stimulus is non-painful, normal somatic receptors are the first to act. If it is a painful stimulation, nociceptors are the first to fire up.

This process includes several steps:

1. Point of origin or contact with stimulus- the point of origin can be mechanical such as cuts, pressures, abrasions and pressure. It can also be chemically inflicted like burns.

2. Reception – It is a process where the nerve ending senses the stimulus.

3. Transmission – When nerve endings sense the stimulus, they transmit the signal to the central nervous system through a series of neurons.

4. Perception – This is where the brain receives the signal for further processing and action.

When you cut your hand, there are several factors that contribute to your perception of pain. First is the mechanical stimulation of the sharp object that cut you. Your cells are damaged and they release potassium. This is why you feel the intense sharp pain at the moment of injury. Then Prostaglandins, histamines and bradykinins from the immune cells invade the area during inflammation. This is the stage where your body is protecting you from the foreign stimulus. You will experience a longer dull ache or numbing feeling along the affected area.

Nociceptor neurons travel in peripheral sensory nerves. The signals are relayed from the free nerve endings at the layer of the skin. These signals are sent to the spinal cord through the dorsal roots. They synapse on the neurons within the spinal cord segment and also two or three segments below and above the point of entry. This is basically the reason why it is sometimes difficult to locate the location of the pain in the body especially when the damage is internal.

Secondary neurons then transmit the signal upward through the spinothalamic tract. The signal travels from the spinothalamic tract to the medulla (brain's system) and ends in the thalamus, which is the central relaying center of the brain. Some neurons also send signal to the medulla's reticular receptors which control the physical behavior.

Once the signal is processed in the brain, some signals will pass through the motor cortex, to the spinal cord then down to the motor nerves. These impulses cause muscle contractions that make you move your hand away from the object.

What are the types of pain?

There are different types of pain. Neuroscientists and physicians classify pain in three ways:

1. Acute pain- This is a type of pain which is inflicted to the body. An injury to the body like a cut or burn causes an acute pain in the affected area. It warns of potential damage and compels action from the brain. It can develop slowly or quickly. Depending on the type of injury and the intensity of the damage, pain can last up to a few minutes to a year. When the wound starts to heal however, acute pain goes away.

2. Chronic pain – It is a persistent kind of pain. It does not require your body to respond unlike acute pain. Chronic pain still persists even when the trauma has been healed. It lasts longer than six months. An example of a chronic pain is a migraine.

3. Cancer/malignant pain – This is a kind of pain associated with tumors. It is somehow associated with chronic pain; however, cancer pain is …

Check out the rest of "Guide to Pain Management: How to Achieve Pain Relief and Live Pain Free for Life" on Amazon.

Or go to: http://amzn.to/1eP7QRh

Check Out My Other Books

Below you'll find some of my other books that are popular on Amazon and Kindle as well. You can visit my author page on Amazon to see other work done by me. Alternatively, you can simply search for these titles on the Amazon website to find them.

Pain Management Guide: How to Achieve Pain Relief and Live Pain Free for Life

Fibromyalgia Book Guide: How to Successfully Live with Fibromyalgia and Recipes for the Fibromyalgia Diet

One Last Thing...

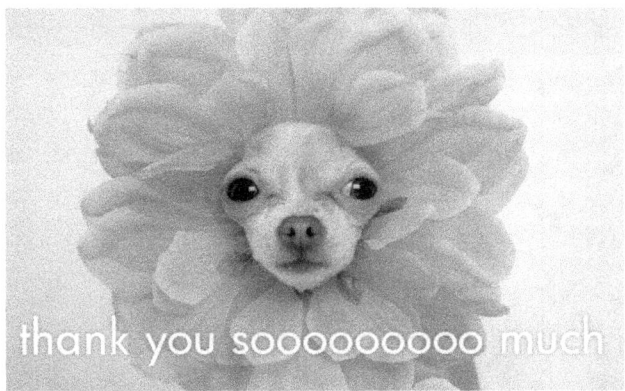

Source: Wikipedia

If you believe that this book is worth sharing, would you please take the time to let others know how it affected your life? If it turns out to make a difference in the lives of others, they will be forever grateful to you, as will I.